Copyright

CLAIRE HUNTER

Break the Diet Habit

I'm on a crusade against diets.

I've had enough of the perpetual lies fed to people who are earnestly trying to improve their own well being.

- That there are quick "fixes".
- That not losing weight as fast as someone else on the same plan means YOU aren't trying hard enough.
- That putting the weight back on again is somehow YOUR failure, and not a built in part of the business plan that depends upon your continued custom.
- That achieving a healthy, balanced body should be uncomfortable.
- That deprivation is healthy.
- That exercise should be painful or gruelling.
- That your body in its current state is so awful that it necessitates "correcting" in the shortest possible time regardless of the impact on your physical or mental health.
- That there are tricks or hacks that will magically cause your body to change for good.

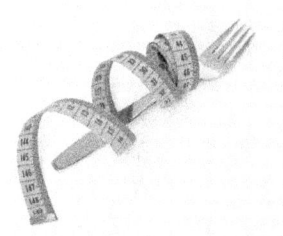

These ideas are demoralising, belittling and make committed, genuinely hard working people feel stranded and helpless.

What if I told you that nobody maintaining lifelong healthy body composition is doing it by using the "rules" and regimens set out by commercial diets and weight loss clubs?

What if I told you that even if your fat mass is much greater than your ideal goal, you don't need to suffer and sacrifice to get there? Instead, providing you are willing to apply a little consistency and patience, you can simply live as if you were there already and allow your body to catch up.

No fads, no quick fixes, no shame, no failure, no counting, just good living through gentle introduction of achievable habits.

What's so different about Free Living Fitness?

We are going to work on building habits, in your diet, lifestyle and exercise, that will lead to a sustainable improvement in your fitness.

Why am I talking about fitness and not weight loss?

Fitness is not just about jumping jacks, it's actually about a whole range of factors, specifically:

- Physical

- Mental and emotional
- Medical (this is not something we will be tackling directly, but will be influenced by the others)
- Nutritional
- Social

Many weight loss programmes take into account only one factor of physical fitness (body composition, or simply body mass), neglecting or even damaging the others. Our aim here is to produce positive effects on all areas.

In practice this means:

- Building dietary habits that support good, balanced nutrition.
- Fitting your fitness plan around your family, social and work life.
- Motivating through positive means, not through shame.
- Building a positive relationship with your body.
- Making habits easy to apply, avoiding time consuming or obsessive tracking.
- Aiming for healthy body composition, which means muscle gain and a healthy body fat percentage.
- Using exercise as a means to have fun and interact with others.
- Improving cardiovascular fitness, strength, stamina and co-ordination, not just burning calories.
- Looking at the bigger picture, not just the numbers on the scale.

I'm not going to promise you dramatic, fast weight loss. You've been promised that before and I suspect that the fact you are here reading this means it didn't go so well for you. So let's try something new.

Some people will experience fairly fast changes, I have a client who lost visible weight within 2 weeks of implementing just one of the nutrition habits, because it hit their biggest barrier to loss just right. But this is a journey towards balance and synchrony in your body, a daily practice that you have the rest of your life to work on. It might be challenging at times, but I know you can do this, for a survivor of the dieting world it's going to be a breeze.

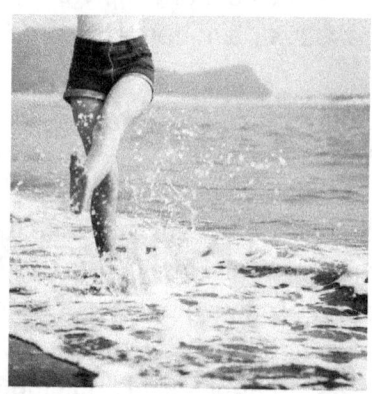

Introducing the habits

People are often surprised when they ask me for weight loss or fitness performance advice and I start talking about anything other than diet and exercise.

After all, didn't I say it was just about calories in vs calories out?

Well it is, but your body's ability to use calories, or digest calories, or even the mechanisms that control your understanding of where that balance lies are affected by some key factors.

If you have been trying to lose weight, and feel like you are doing the right things but it still isn't happening, it's likely that one of these other core factors is coming into play, so we are going to be working on those too. This is how it breaks down.

Diet

Your body mass is effectively controlled by the amount of food you eat. Or more specifically the calories you consume. You eat more than you use, you put on mass, you eat less, you lose mass. But we can't take that as the whole story, because "mass" is not just "fat mass". Mass is also your 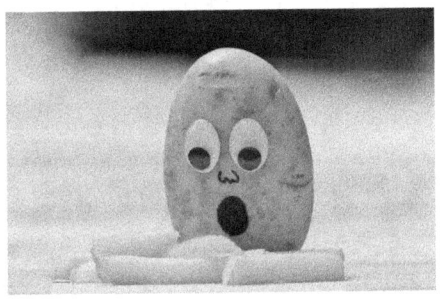 muscle mass and your bone mass, as well as a few other factors, like water. Diets that cut calories (often dramatically), but don't consider exercise, lifestyle or the quality of those calories will lose you mass, but the number on the scales means nothing if you are actually fuelling yourself by consuming your own muscle.

The composition of your body is determined by the quality of your diet (as well as your exercise). So we are going to be focusing as much as possible on eating whole, unprocessed foods, lean protein and generally keeping the quality high to give your body the building blocks it needs to be strong and healthy.

You have a very good built-in calorie monitoring system. Hunger will tell you when you need to eat more, or when you have had enough. Many people have stopped listening to their hunger and satiety, or interpret other signals as a cue to eat. We are going to relearn how to listen and respond appropriately to the needs of our bodies.

Exercise

Exercise isn't just about workouts, it's about keeping active on a regular basis, throughout your day. Ideally you need to be moving and active for at least 30 minutes a day, at least 10 minutes at a time - but if you can fit in more, even better.

There's a lot of myths and debate about what kind of exercise is best. You need to be doing cardiovascular exercise (cardio for short) for the health of your heart and lungs. It's also a really useful way to train your muscles to access their fuel efficiently so you can exercise harder. Finding time for long duration, steady state cardio can be difficult, so I'm giving you some High Intensity Interval Training (HIIT) which blasts through a lot of calories in a shorter time while challenging your cardiovascular system.

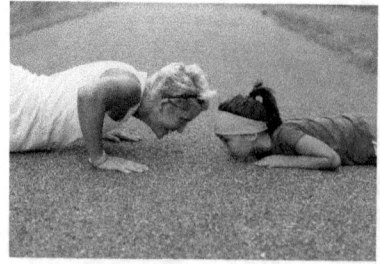

One thing that is becoming very clear, is that resistance (weight) training is really important for general health and also for fat loss. Women and men benefit from the same kinds of training (makes sense, muscles are muscles after all, women's are smaller - but just as powerful gram for gram). Resistance training improves your muscle which boosts your metabolism, gives you shape, makes you feel strong, move easier and generally feel more awesome.

Resistance workouts should be challenging - there is no point in lifting a weight you can lift for more than 20 reps without a break. If you don't have access to a gym, that's fine, you can use bodyweight exercises which are just as challenging, and maybe some resistance bands. These start out at fairly low resistance, but you can buy bands which have up to 100kg resistance. You don't need to buy dumbells and bands are super cheap (not the 100kg ones, but you won't need those and they are still cheaper than weights).

The Free Living Fitness Movement Programme was written to complement this one. It takes you from couch to active and it comes with both cardio and resistance workouts. Some are for gym based training (or require some equipment) and some for home, so you can choose to train exclusively at one location, or mix it up a bit. They are progressive, and workouts are ascribed to particular weeks. I've kept the movement and lifestyle programmes separate however, because some folks have their own, preferred exercise, and that's just fine. In fact it's great.

The entire ethos of Free Living Fitness is that you should do what feels best for you.

Sleep

Sleep is one of the most important factors that affects our health and fitness. If you are tired, you will consume more calories than you need as your hunger signals are confused. Tired people are less active, so expend less calories. That's not news, everyone knows that the best follow up to a late night is a day of lying on the sofa eating junk food!

Sleep is also the time when your body recovers from your workouts, building new muscle and repairing damage. Fit healthy people sleep well. People who train hard and don't sleep suffer from fatigue and don't get the results they should do. So we will be implementing some habits to help you sleep better too.

Stress Management

If sleep is one thing that will sap your willpower and make you struggle to eat appropriately, stress has to come a close second. Stress is a major factor for people who struggle with hedonic eating (eating for reasons other than real hunger). Stress hormones can also cause upset to our metabolism, when they are around all the time rather than simply when they are needed.

Stress isn't always a bad thing. It is a useful physiological response to danger in our environment. Some people thrive on stress. Those guys who use the changes in their body as a deadline approaches to become more focused and productive, or athletes who recognise their nerves and use the adrenaline time warp to turn out perfect form and performance.

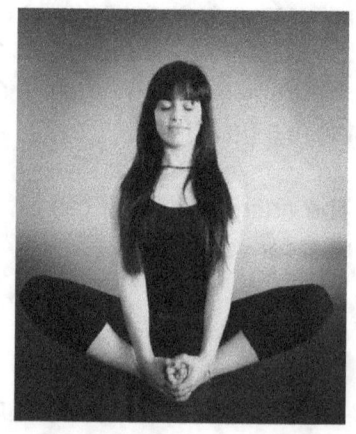

Stress is a bit like having an elephant working at a building site. Super useful if you can harness him and get some heavy work done, a completely destructive nightmare if he is allowed to run free without purpose.

So managing stress and keeping it tame is going to be part of our plan too.

Mindset

Often when we are out of sync with our bodies, the work that needs to happen is not just about changing our bodies.

I don't believe it is possible to motivate healthful choices and positive changes from a place of shame or negativity, it's certainly not easy. Many people struggle to lose weight or keep exercising because negative feelings about their bodies lead them to feel that they don't deserve it, or they can't do it, or their relationship with their body is so unforgiving that even if they were to get into incredible shape, they still wouldn't feel happy with their body or comfortable in their skin.

To that end let me explain that my primary goal on this plan is to help you to feel more comfortable in your skin. By feeling brighter, functioning better, looking fabulous and also being proud of what your body is, and is capable of in itself.

It's beyond my scope to go in depth with the issues that lead people to become detached and out of love for their bodies, but we will be working on building a healthy mindset and appreciating our bodies along the way.

Your lifestyle plan

In order to maintain good health and, ultimately, your goal weight, you are going to need to make a long term commitment to some lifestyle changes. None of these will be uncomfortable in the long term, this isn't a lifelong diet! But they may be challenging to implement as it is natural to want to resist any change to your established routine.

You may well discover that you have some quite strong attachments to your current ways. You might be surprised at the ferocity of your emotional objection to changes that are objectively fairly simple and logically better for you. That's perfectly normal and when it happens, it's worth stepping back and taking a look at where that response is coming from.

The first thing to realise however is that you cannot expect different results from the same routine. You want change? You have to make some changes. It's your choice. But you do get to do this at your own pace. There is no point trying to make dozens of changes all at once, it feels stifling and overwhelming. So we are going to take it slow, one habit at a time.

Your plan works in phases, you'll spend at least a week on a phase, practicing the habits until they start to feel normal. I would expect you to take 2 weeks on most phases, that's a good timeframe for a new habit, but some of the habits will come easier, or be similar to your current lifestyle choices. Some will be trickier and I would encourage you to stay in those phases until they feel right and natural to you -

even if it takes a little bit longer. Some of the habits are consistent through multiple phases.

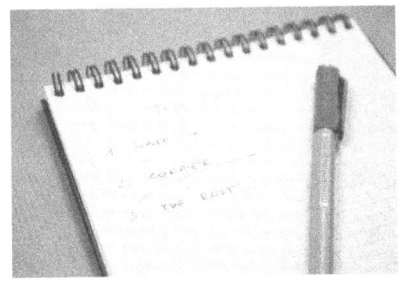

For every phase of the plan, I'm going to give you a checklist. It contains 3 habits that I would like you to practice daily. Work at all of them, you win if you get them checked off every day. Give yourself a big pat on the back. If you miss one, don't worry, it's not the end of the world, you can try again tomorrow. Consistency is getting your habits 80% of the time, that gives you 4 checkboxes leeway every week, and you're still winning!

Not every one of the habits is going to suit everyone. That's fine. I'm not asking you to maintain each and every one of these for life. What I would like you to do is give them a good go. Make sure you can maintain the habit consistently for 2 weeks, and see what you learn from that. You might learn you are capable of something you thought you weren't, you might even find it becomes easy and comfortable. You might learn something about your previous habits, for instance cutting out high calorie drinks might help highlight to you quite how much you were previously relying on them, and how much you might be able to cut back. On the other hand you might just discover a tool that suddenly makes managing your health a whole lot easier.

I'm providing you with a grid in every chapter, which you can copy and stick somewhere prominent, to record your habits every day. There's also another copy in the appendix at the back.

You may also wish to invest in the Free Living Fitness Daily Planner. I designed it to work with this programme, helping you keep track of your progress and stay accountable, with a page per day journal.

Phase 1

This is the part where we lay down the foundations of all the things we will be working on!

Nutrition

Your goal in this phase is to record a "food and mood" diary. We won't be keeping this up throughout, unless you find it enjoyable and useful, but this week is all about being mindful of what you are eating.

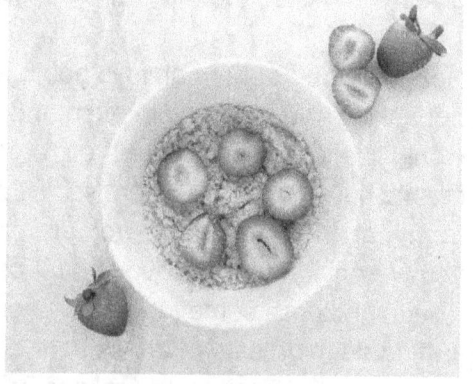

You are going to make a note of what you are eating and when. I'd also like you to note down how hungry you were before you ate, and after you finished. 0 is wanting to eat your own arm, 5 is stuffed and uncomfortable. Then I'd like you to make a rough note of your mood in general.

We aren't going to judge, or start trying to make major changes just yet, just get a bearing on how things lie. I'd like you to think about why you chose to eat when and what you did. Were you hungry, or bored?

Did you eat more than you needed to feel satisfied, or perhaps less? When did you start feeling hungry again after finishing a meal?

This kind of mindfulness is really important. We tend to become detached from our true hunger. We eat out of habit, obligation, social pressure, emotion and for all kinds of other reasons that have little to do with our bodies' need for fuel. We learn to ignore our satiety as children told to clear our plates, and to ignore our hunger as adults trying to lose weight. The greatest part of our work here will be to reconnect with our hunger, as a useful tool for understanding our needs.

So our only goal right now is to observe, however, if you feel like you would like to get a head start on eating a bit better, try these little tips to be going on with:

- Hydrate well, drink a glass of water every time you eat or exercise
- Eat single portions at one time. A portion of protein is a palmful (or a deck of cards) carbs is a fistfull, veg is a handful, fatty food like cheese and nuts is a portion the size of your thumb. Packaged foods come labelled with a suggested portion size. If you eat a single portion and still feel unsatisfied, take another, but don't put 2 on your plate and feel obliged to eat them.
- Eat when you are hungry in the belly (not the head) and stop when you feel comfortably satisfied, not stuffed.
- Eat a portion of protein 3-4 times a day.
- Aim for 5 portions of fruit and veg.
- Try to fill your meals with whole foods, as close to their natural state as possible.

We will do some proper work on all of these in later phases, so you don't need to have these down right now, but forewarned is forearmed!

Activity.

There's a lot of argument about the most effective exercise for weight loss. Ultimately it's much of a muchness. HIIT is great because you fit a lot of activity into a short space of time, but it doesn't actually use more calories than steady cardio for an appropriate duration. In truth, exercise actually makes a fairly small dent in your daily calorie expenditure.

Exercise IS super important. Building muscle gives us strength to move around in our bodies comfortably. Developed muscles give our bodies shape and firmness, which is nice. Increased muscle mass does improve metabolism and exercise is generally great for well being, mental health and energy levels. The fitness you gain through exercise makes it easier to be active the rest of your day.

Because what actually burns the most calories isn't that half hour of intensive cardio, it's the hours of gentle activity in between. In fact people, but especially women, are really good at "making up" calories expended during intense exercise, by being less active for the rest of the day, without even noticing it!

We call this kind of movement NEAT (Non Exercise Activity Thermogenesis!) But what you need to know is that moving around and being active throughout your day will do you a lot more good, both in terms of health and weight management, than sitting on the couch all day then doing an aerobics class in the evening.

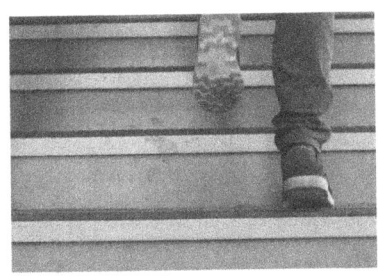

Activity could be walking, housework, gardening anything like that. Being more active could involve taking a stroll on your lunch break, getting off the bench and playing with your kids in the park, taking the stairs (that old chestnut...). It might mean getting up from your desk and walking over to a colleague's office instead of emailing a question. Lots of little things add up.

We will work on these gradually and your exercise programme is going to help you feel stronger, fitter, more energetic and motivated to move more in your everyday life.

Your first activity goal is simple, it's the general recommendation for activity, which is to spend a total of 30 minutes a day being moderately active in periods of at least 10 minutes at a time.

You can handle this. 3, 10 minute walks a day. 10 minutes vacuuming and a 20 minute stroll. Or go all out and count an exercise class. I don't mind what you do, as long as you are moving continuously and it is slightly more than your usual level of activity. Get moving, tick it off the list. Done.

Wellbeing

Some people are great at managing their stress, some people not so much. This week's habit is to introduce 5 minutes of

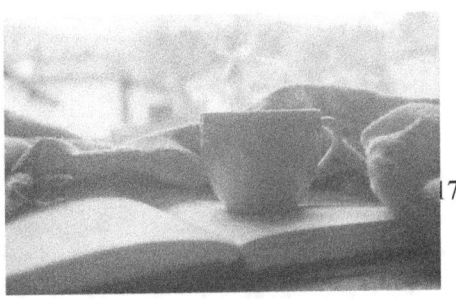

brain defrag into your day, every day.

It's up to you how you do this. Lots of people enjoy a bit of meditation, you don't have to do anything fancy, just sit quietly and observe your breathing, take note, but let go of any feelings in your body, or noises from your surroundings. Mindfulness meditation is also great exercise for your willpower; by acknowledging distractions but making the decision not to engage with them you are rehearsing for making tough decisions later. There are various guided meditations available to support this. Or you could just do some deep breathing exercises for 5 minutes.

Some people are organisers (or find lack of clarity stressful) and find taking time to write a list of the things they need to take care of helps, by getting it out of their head and onto paper. Or perhaps try keeping a gratitude journal and use your 5 minutes to write down a few good things about your day.

You might have an activity that helps you manage stress, like art, taking a bath, or walking in nature. In which case your goal is to do this on a daily basis, even if it's just for a very brief time.

I filmed this savasana sequence, which is a good place to start if this is new to you Try it out, it takes less than 10 minutes.
https://youtu.be/Djr1fZ4c4GY

We won't track your stress management habit throughout the programme, but you will feel and perform much better if you keep it up.

So that's your plan!

You can start working on this straight away. I have deliberately separated the exercise and lifestyle habits in this programme to allow you to work on each at your own pace. You might even feel that right now, the activity set out here is enough and you want to hold out on bringing in any workouts until you feel a little fitter, and that's absolutely fine. You might find that you progress faster through the lifestyle changes than the exercise, or vice versa. That's fine too. This is your journey and there really is no need to rush.

Food and mood diary

Try to put down everything you eat at roughly the correct time of day. Rate your hunger before and after you ate on a scale of 1-5.
0 = painfully hungry, trying not to eat the cat 1 = stomach pangs 2 = a bit peckish, grumbling belly 3 = comfortable 4= satisfied 5 = uncomfortably full

Take a note of your mood throughout the day, just write the first word that comes to mind.

	6-9am	9-12	12-3pm	3-6pm	6-9pm	9-12pm
Day 1 Food						

Hunger before/ after						
Mood						

Your Phase 1 checklist

Day	1	2	3	4	5	6	7
Updated my food and mood diary							
Completed 30 minutes of activity today							
5 minutes stress management							

Phase 2

Nutrition

The nutrition habit for this phase is a great one. I've found it makes a huge difference to clients who can get this one down. It's simple:

Eat 3 or 4 times a day.

Easy! In between those times you can have drinks, like tea, water etc, but not milky or sugary drinks. We don't do snacks. We just do meals, good proper meals that fill you up for 4-5 hours.

This might be a bit different to what you have been told before, a lot of diets advocate eating "little and often", but we know those diets aren't working for us, so we are going to try something else. I'm not just throwing spaghetti at the wall and seeing what sticks either, there's solid science behind this.

SCIENCE!

When you eat, your insulin levels rise, in response to both carbohydrates and protein. When there are high levels of insulin in your system, your body won't fuel itself on stored fat. Why would it when there is plenty of fuel in the form of glucose, right there in your blood? You also don't use your fat stores when your carbohydrate stores (glycogen in your muscles and liver) are plentiful. If you eat at intervals of under about 3 hours, your insulin levels keep getting topped up and your glycogen stores are plentiful, so your body doesn't need to start unpacking that fat, and over time, it can get less efficient at it. You'll notice this if you are the sort of person who suddenly gets a raging hunger out of nowhere, around 3 hours after you have eaten. Your body isn't switching to fat oxidation efficiently and your blood glucose suffers as a result.

That's why this habit is important.

[Side note, the above applies to an average, healthy person; anyone with a diagnosed or suspected metabolic or blood sugar regulation disorder may react differently to this sort of thing - if that's you, you need to be talking to a dietitian who is able to offer a suitable diet plan].

In addition, it has been shown that people who eat more than 4 times a day generally consume more calories than those who eat in 3-4 sittings. Makes sense. There's a limit to how much you can eat in one go!

I first came across this habit through Georgia Fear's Lean Habits (which I would definitely recommend for anyone who wants to get into the nitty gritty of their nutrition, or find out more about the science behind all this stuff.) Many of the habits which she uses, I was already implementing with myself and my clients, but not this one. It makes a lot of sense, the science and the supporting evidence is solid. I felt I had to use this one to help my clients.

But... I don't ever ask a client to do something I haven't done myself, which meant that even though I was pretty happy with my nutrition plan, I needed to give this a go for a couple of weeks at least.

I was surprised by my reaction to this realisation. The thought of eliminating between-meal eating, even if I got 4 meals and they got to be big, satisfying meals, made me genuinely ANGRY!

I had to take myself aside and have a serious think about why this was such a big deal for me. I guess I really like snacks! I think often we carry an emotional attachment to certain ways of eating. Elevenses reminds me of being at home with my mum, afternoon snacks with my children after school are a nice time to reconnect, snacking while watching a film in the evening is a lovely treat.

I gave it a go anyway and this is what I found:

- It is immensely satisfying to eat a full meal, instead of a slightly cut down one, which you can do if you aren't eating 5-6 times a day.I'm eating 6-800 calories at a sitting, instead of 3-600. I don't get up from a meal unfulfilled, I don't feel hungry again an hour after breakfast.
- You can have your "snacks" if you make them part of your meal. I often eat fruit, yoghurt, milky coffee, protein shakes etc as "dessert" rather than keeping them for later, and they are just as good!
- It's actually a bit of a relief not having to carry snacks around with me all the time in case I get hungry.
- I don't have to plan multiple meals, or pack them and carry them.
- I don't have to shop for specific snack foods, which tend to be relatively expensive.
- Considering my "4th meal" as a meal and not a snack enables me to eat properly when I need to. So if I come home after an evening workout and need to eat, I'm not eating a small snack, then still feeling hungry and eating another small snack, and another... I'm making myself a small meal (like eggs and toast) from the outset, feeling more full, eating healthier foods and often less calorie intake.

I like it. I started implementing it with clients as soon as I realised this. They liked it, and had some incredible results, and that is why I am asking you to give it a go for a couple of weeks and see how you like it!

You can plan for 3 or 4 meals at set times, or switch it around depending on your day.You can keep your 4th meal as a roving snack depending on your schedule. It might be a latte and something to eat in a coffee shop when you meet a friend, or an "early tea" because you are eating out later. It might be a light meal after an evening workout, or planned snacks watching a movie. Or you might drop it on some days because 3 feel like enough. You can master your habit while still allowing yourself flexibility, and that makes it easy to stick with.

Activity

Keep working on those 30 minutes a day. Perhaps you can find a new way to do it?

Wellbeing

Many of us talk to ourselves in ways that we would never dream of talking to another person, even in ways we would never allow another person to talk to us. By doing this we damage ourselves, chipping away at our self esteem every single day.

Negative self-talk is not just a compulsive habit that we build up ourselves. It is reinforced by a culture that encourages us to be self-deprecating, where demonstrably feeling good about ourselves is labelled as conceited, prideful or vain.

We are going to start gently. For many people thinking positively about our bodies can be too great a leap, so we are going to start work on drowning out our inner critic with neutral thoughts.

Your goal is to take a moment every day, maybe check yourself out in the mirror, maybe you don't.

You can simply say to yourself (aloud if you can, not if that feels uncomfortable):

"This is my body, as it is right now"

Without judgement or emotion. You might feel you can add "and that's OK" or something if you feel you are ready for that, but you don't need to, right now, we are looking for simple acceptance and ownership.

You can use the same statement every day, or you can think of other, neutral statements that sit well with you. It might feel a bit odd at first, but that's part of the point - if you aren't used to thinking positive, or even neutral things about your body, it's definitely something to work at.

Your Phase 2 checklist

Day	1	2	3	4	5	6	7
Ate 3-4 times in the day							
30 minutes walking or light activity							
Neutral self talk							

Phase 3

Nutrition

Hopefully by now you are getting a handle on eating 3-4 times a day, and that probably means that you are getting used to feeling real belly hunger and being OK with that.

Many people have a dysfunctional relationship with their hunger. A history of deprivation, or abundance; eating disorders, plate clearing habits, diet "rules" (like eating every 3 hours) that gloss over our natural self regulation. There's all kinds of reasons why we might ignore or fear our hunger.

But our hunger is how our bodies speak to us to let us know when, how much, even what to eat. Tuning into these subtle messages is the key to eating appropriately to our needs without counting, tracking or arbitrary rules.

Our next nutrition habit is listening to our hunger.

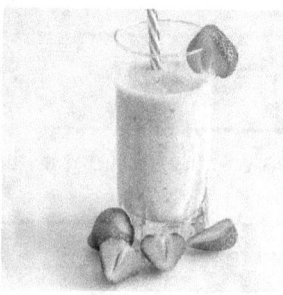

You'll likely be aware that you have both hunger and appetite. Hunger is the signal that your body needs to eat, appetite is your drive to eat.

If you've ever been recovering from an illness and felt that stomach growling hunger but still not felt like eating, then you've experienced hunger without appetite. And pretty much everyone has been in that place where they have wanted to eat but not needed to.

Distinguishing between hunger cues and appetite is a really useful skill for weight management. Many people overeat because they are responding to sensations other than hunger with eating - this builds into a habit to the point where it gets hard to tell the difference.

So in this phase, **when you feel hungry, try to wait for 30 minutes before you eat**. If you are experiencing false hunger, coming from boredom, emotional state or habit, it is likely that will pass in about 20 minutes if you ignore it and focus on something else (that's important, if you obsess and count down you are still going to want to eat - but there is still value in holding off and practicing sitting with that discomfort). If you are still hungry, in the belly not the head, after 30 minutes, then it's probably time to eat.

I'd also like you to try not to wait too long after 30 minutes - if you get too hungry (remember 0 on the food and mood diary?) then you are likely to overeat.

There's an art to eating enough at one meal to carry you through to 30 minutes before the next mealtime before you feel hungry, but this is a work in progress, it's OK to miss the mark while you are finding your feet, or at any point thereafter!

If you have had problems with hunger in the past, perhaps it is an emotionally loaded sensation, you might feel uneasy about spending a long period in this state to start with. In this case, build up slowly, try 5 minutes. If you survive 5 minutes, maybe try a little longer next time. Slowly let yourself realise that hunger isn't a dangerous or urgent sensation, it's simply information letting you know where your body is at.

Activity

Keep up your 30 minutes a day, but now we are going to add in a new habit.

Move often. Studies show that moving regularly throughout the day is more effective that bunching all your non-exercise activity into a solid chunk and sitting the rest of the time. It improves your mood and it reduces your food cravings!

So set yourself a reminder on your phone, or sit an hourglass on your desk. Both the Apple watch and Fitbit have regular movement goals/reminders built in.

Then once an hour, stand up, take a 5 minute walk somewhere - the bathroom, the photocopier, the water cooler, go look out of the window. If you can't do that, try standing up where you are, do some ankle circles, point and flex your toes, get the blood flowing a bit (try looking up DVT prevention exercises for travel - easy movement you can do discreetly while seated).

Aim to break up your day with 6 or more short movement bouts, however that works best for you. And keep up the 30 minutes of movement in bouts of at least 10 minutes.

Wellbeing

Your sleep time is really crucial. Sleep deprivation can cause all kinds of health issues, and many of us get by on suboptimal sleep.

Sleeping organises your body on all kinds of levels, it regulates hormones (including those that control your metabolism and hunger), allows you to process stress and gives your body time to recover and repair itself. Without enough sleep, stress, fatigue, overeating, injury, irritability and reduced cognitive function start to become problematic.

This week's goal is to allocate yourself enough time to sleep.

Figure out what time you need to get up in the morning, and count back 8 hours. Your aim is to be in bed, ready to sleep by that time, in order that you give yourself the chance to sleep for around 7 ½ hours.

You might not go to sleep straight away. That's fine. You are simply bookmarking that section of the day for sleep, not for work, or watching TV or any of the other things that might keep you up late of an evening.

Bedtime means in bed, dressed for bed, with all your tasks for the day dealt with, or at least put aside deliberately (maybe in the form of a list for tomorrow). You can take a warm non-caffeinated, non-alcoholic drink with you. You can read until you feel sleepy, but try to avoid electronics. If you are a phone addict it might be worth keeping it out of reach.

Your Phase 3 checklist

Day	1	2	3	4	5	6	7
Waited 30 minutes hungry before eating							
Moved around for 5 minutes 6 times during the day							
Went to bed on time							

Phase 4

Congratulations for getting this far! So far you have learned some habits that help you to be more aware of what you are eating, and why. You have also learned some strategies for reducing your calorie input - feeling your hunger and eating fewer, but more substantial meals. Those are really useful skills and I hope they are starting to feel comfortable. Now we are going to make it even easier, by starting to look at what you are eating.

Nutrition

The next nutrition habit looks at protein. Whenever I look at a food diary, the most common and glaring problem is a lack of protein.

To get sciencey, in order to avoid malnutrition, most people need to take about 18% of their calories as protein, which is roughly 0.8g of dietary protein per kilo bodyweight. That means a 70kg, sedentary, individual needs about 56g of protein a day - about 10 eggs or just less than 2 chicken breasts! But that's just to avoid diseases of malnutrition. Research shows us that a diet of around 30% calories as protein has notable benefits to the metabolism. That could be twice as much as the minimum!

Food is not just fuel, it's also communication, a way of instructing your body on how to work. Protein stimulates the hormones in our body that make us feel satiated. That is to say, when you eat protein with a meal, you feel fuller for longer. Eating a good portion of protein with every meal will help you go for longer before that hunger kicks in, bolstering your existing work.

Enough protein in your diet also helps prevent your body from using the protein in your muscles for fuel, and that's good, because you need those muscles!

Your goal this phase is to introduce a dense source of lean protein with 3 meals a day. We aren't going to count grams or track macros or any of those things, just making an effort to include something is enough for now, but if you aren't sure if something is high in protein, look at the label, you're looking for 15-25g of protein in a suggested portion. A portion of protein dense food is around the size of your palm or a pack of playing cards.

Here are some tips for including proteins with conventional meals:

Breakfast
Add a fromage frais or icelandic style yoghurt (10-15g)
Use granary or seeded bread instead of white (around 5-6g a slice)
Add smoked salmon to toast or scrambled eggs.
Add 2 eggs (12g)

Choose a high protein granola (extra points for buckwheat which is a complete protein)
Add turkey bacon or lean meat slices.

Lunch
Add cottage cheese.
Add in some chicken or fish (extra points for oily fish with omega 3 oils)
Eat a protein bar for dessert.
Top your salad with edamame beans and sugar snap peas.

Dinner
Lean meat (no skin no fat).
Soy protein
Quorn
Replace or partially substitute rice for quinoa.
Use high protein vegetables, consider partially replacing starchy carbs with beans/lentils.

Doing it vegan

If you eat meat or dairy, it's not hard to get lean, complete proteins into your diet. A really nice lazy option is to just add in more chicken breast, cottage cheese and thick yoghurts! Vegan protein sources are available and it is entirely possible to eat a high protein plant based diet. It just takes a little thought. If you are going down this road consider making at least one of your protein portions a

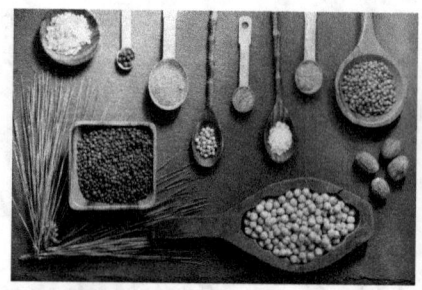

complete protein (buckwheat, quinoa or soy), and have a look on the internet for high protein vegan recipes, there are many out there.

Try to mix up your protein sources, don't just eat one type of bean, eat a few types together, with some peas/lentils and green veg. That will help you get a better range of amino acids and avoid too much starch alongside your protein.

One last tip, which goes as much for non-vegans as vegans - protein tends to naturally occur with fats. This is why I say "lean protein". When you eat chicken, you take the skin off and that's most of the fat gone, but you can't do that with foods like nuts! Nuts are often referred to as high in protein, but if you eat a portion of nuts large enough to provide you with a good dose of protein, you will be eating too much fat and a lot of calories, so keep high calorie protein dense foods like nuts and cheese to "fat" portions, that's a thumb, not a palm! Include nuts in your meals, but make sure you put in other proteins to make the full portion.

Protein supplements

Another way to introduce a portion of protein, without taking on extra calories or other macronutrients, is to look at a protein supplement, usually in the form of a protein powder. You can get plant based and dairy based powders. Some are flavourless and great in smoothies or recipes (vegetable based protein makes a great soup thickener) and some come flavoured and prepped ready to just add water (or milk) for a shake drink.

My advice for supplements generally is to always get your nutrition from real, whole food sources wherever possible. If however you are struggling to add in protein to your breakfast, or want something easy on the go, it would be reasonable to add in a portion of protein powder to your day.

Activity

Keep working on moving regularly through the day, this ones a good one, so we will get it really cemented in.

Wellbeing

We are going to keep working on this bedtime malarkey, because I know this one takes persistent practice and slips easily.

I'm going to take a moment here to consider electronics. I've already suggested that once bedtime hits, there are no electronics (TV, phones, laptops etc) and that if you are not sleeping you could perhaps read, meditate, colour etc. The reason for this is that electronic devices give off a lot of light on the 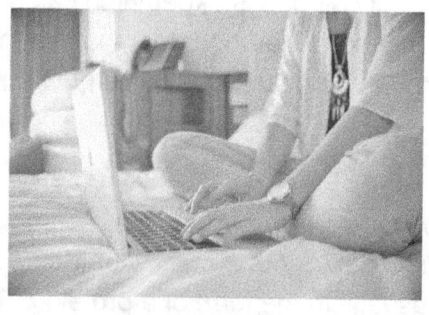 blue end of the spectrum - they imitate daylight. This kind of light tricks your brain and stops you from producing the hormones you need for a good night's sleep.

Sleep experts will tell you to put away the screens at least an hour before bed, ideally several hours before.

I understand how hard this can be, especially if the evening is your best time to get some peace, enjoy some TV, gaming or social media. It might even be the best time for you to get some work done at your computer. In this case I'm going to suggest you look at a blue light filter programme. I use f.lux on my laptop and an app on my phone. These shift the colour of the light produced by your device, usually switching automatically at a given time. It makes your screen look slightly orange, but you do get used to it. Unless you are working on a colour dependent project, like photo editing, the function is much the same.

Either way, those electronics go away at bedtime. Any post bedtime, pre sleeping activity needs to be old school and blue light free.

Your Phase 4 checklist

Day	1	2	3	4	5	6	7
Ate 3 portions of protein							
Moved around for 5 minutes 6 times during the day							
Practiced bedtime routine							

Phase 5

Brilliant! You are nearly halfway now, so I hope you are getting into the swing of things. That said, just before halfway always seems to be the point where motivation starts to dip, be mindful of this. Remind yourself how far you have come and how well you are doing.

Nutrition

This phase we are going to work on satiety. So far you've been giving yourself space to get hungry, feeling the hunger and eaten more protein to give you a bit longer before you are hungry. You have achieved mastery of hunger! Now it's time to master satiety!

A really common reason for overeating is that we often eat mindlessly, or so fast that our physiology doesn't get the chance to register that we've eaten enough until it's too late. Our bodies recognise that we've eaten in a number of ways, from the stretching of the stomach to detecting the presence of nutrition molecules as they are absorbed. When we eat fast we have to rely on the stomach "fullness" as an indicator, but that's not very accurate, especially when we are eating calorie dense foods or if we've conditioned ourselves to ignore it. We have to give our systems time to register.

So your goal this phase is to **eat slowly and mindfully - and stop when you feel satisfied.**

Start by choosing one meal a day to work on. Check the clock and aim to take 15 minutes to eat that meal. There are a number of ways you can slow yourself down if you are a natural dinner-inhaler. Try setting down your fork between bites, or not loading your fork until you have swallowed the last mouthful. Take time to appreciate and enjoy each bite.

You are aiming to eat until you are satisfied, but not stuffed. That's a 4 on your hunger scale.

Now we have a bigger picture, you eat when you are at a 1-2 (hungry, but not famished) and until you are a 4 (satisfied, not stuffed). That's the sweet spot. If you are trying to lose weight, the difference you need may be just a couple of mouthfuls less - about "80% full".

Activity

By now you should be a total expert at keeping yourself moving through the day, so now let's get ourselves set up correctly for every day.

A really great movement coach once said that if you start the day with a routine that puts your body into good movement patterns, every step from thereon is therapy.

The Wellbeing goal in this phase is about getting up on time, so let's give you a great way to start the day.

Take a couple of minutes first thing to do some mobility exercises that set you up right. You could do some stretches, a short yoga flow or a selection of the stability exercises that you find most beneficial for your body.

I've also put together a short flow here:

- Start by opening your hands really big, then bunching up into fists for a few cycles. Then circle your wrists/fists in both directions.

- Flex your feet and spread your toes, then point your toes, again for a few cycles, now circle the feet/ankles.
- Turn the head slowly to face over one shoulder, then the other, then back to centre, lift the forehead to the ceiling, throat long, then drop your chin to your chest.
- Stand up and reach to the ceiling super tall. Fold forward, hinging at the hips, and hang there for a moment. Stand up again, keeping the spine neutral, lifting the arms sit back into the hips as if lowering into a chair. Repeat for a couple of rounds.
- Twist the upper body allowing your arms to swing.
- Reach up to the ceiling first one side, then the other, to open up the sides.
- Stand in good posture and take 3 deep, belly breaths.

There's a video example here: https://youtu.be/fL90zDOXlml

Wellbeing

New sleep goal - Don't hit snooze.

Do you have an alarm waking you up in the morning? Do you have the habit of rolling over and snoozing the alarm repeatedly? The half-sleep you are getting during this time is most likely making you feel groggy and slowing you down.

You have 2 options:

1) Leave your alarm set as it is, and just make yourself get up on time. Maybe put your alarm on the other side of the room so you have to get up and switch it off. Then get up and have an extra 10 (20?) minutes to eat a good breakfast, do a little bit of exercise or get some work underway first thing.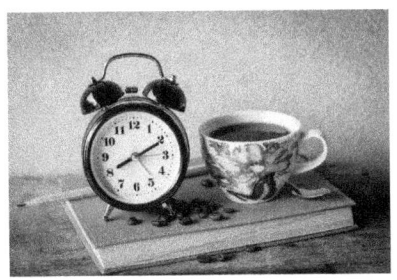

2) Set your alarm for the time you actually get up, and sleep properly until it goes off. Then get up first time, no snooze.

It might take a bit of effort at first, but most people who try this find that they start feeling brighter and clearer on getting up. Starting the day well sets you up for the rest of the day feeling productive and switched on.

Your phase 5 checklist

Day	1	2	3	4	5	6	7
Ate one meal slowly, and stopped when satisfied							
Started the day with movement							
Got up on the first alarm							

Phase 6

Welcome to Phase 6, and congratulations! You made it past the hump!

Nutrition

This nutrition habit is so super basic, but I can almost guarantee you aren't doing it.

It's simple: Drink a glass of water with each meal, and during/after each workout or bout of exercise.

A glass of water is about 250ml, so that's going to be about a litre a day.

"But wait"... I hear you say "am I not supposed to drink 8 glasses of water a day?" Well sure you are, but I bet you aren't and as we always take things in baby steps, this is where we are going to start.

Try a glass with every meal. I don't mind how, you can sip it as you eat, you might find a sip between bites is really helpful with your slowing down habit. Personally I like to down my water. If I leave a glass to sip I'll never finish it, so I tend to fill and drink at the sink and get it over with, usually just before I dish up my food. Some people like to have a water bottle which they keep with them and sip throughout the day. I find this good for hydrating during workouts.

Water balance is really important, it affect so many aspects of your wellbeing that you will likely notice the difference for yourself when you start hydrating consistently.

Drinking before a meal also really helps with mistaking thirst for hunger, which is a common problem.

Activity

We're still pushing the morning flow, this is a great habit, but it needs ingraining into your day so you start to do it automatically on waking.

Wellbeing

So you've been working for a little while on drowning out that negative self talk with positive or neutral observations or statements, that's good work and I'd like you to keep at it.

This phase we are going to introduce a practical element. The habit for this week is to take a little time every day for self care. Do something that makes you feel good and comfortable in yourself, just for yourself every day. It might be taking a bath, or having a pedicure, taking some time to read a book… any of those things you might consider avoiding because you "haven't earned it" or simply because you aren't top priority.

What about something like opening your mail so that pile stops sitting there, silently judging you? Get it done and feel like a boss. Self care is about removing the things that are causing stress and sometimes that means going straight to the cause and sorting it out, so you can relax and not worry about it.

Taking care of your health, through eating well and exercising, is also a form of self-care. And that means it's also easy to let it fall by the wayside if you deprioritise yourself or convince yourself you are not worthy of it. Make it a part of your routine to practice self-care without question.

Your phase 6 checklist

Day	1	2	3	4	5	6	7
Drank a glass of water with each meal and workout							
Started the day with movement							
Daily act of self care							

Phase 7

Phase 7 has arrived, and we are on the home straight! Keep it up!

Nutrition

So far we have focused very much on why and how you eat. With the exception of introducing more protein (which is really to facilitate the "how" by allowing you to feel fuller) we haven't made any changes to **what** you eat. This isn't a mistake at all.

Firstly changing the food that makes up your diet requires changes in how you shop and prepare food, it's a bit of a jolt to your usual lifestyle, and it feels a lot like "dieting".

Secondly. When it comes to weight management, how much you eat (essentially calories) has more impact than what you eat (regardless of what some click-bait internet articles will tell you) and therefore making small changes to your eating patterns in order to eliminate overeating is by my reckoning, the kindest and easiest way to set you up for eating in accordance with your body's needs.

That's not the whole picture. As well as making sure that you meet your energy needs without feeling like you still need to eat more; we have to make sure that you are getting a good balance of all the other things you need to be healthy. Vitamins, minerals and other micronutrients.

Many of these things come from vegetables. They also come from other food sources, but we've nailed them already, so now it is veggie time!

A portion of veg for our purposes is going to be a fistful! Imagine you are at some kind of vegetable buffet but there's no plates left, grab a fistful, or 2 if you like, of veg.

Eat a variety of vegetables. Choose colourful ones, because colour means nutrients. Have some cooked and some raw, because that changes what your body is able to extract from it. For instance raw spinach in your salad is a great source of vitamin C, but steamed spinach is a better source of iron and calcium. You don't have to worry about what comes from where, just eat a mixture of different things.

Your goal is going to be to eat a large portion of veg with each meal, or 3 times a day.

Tips for vegetable eating

When you do your weekly shop, buy in some staple, familiar veg, but also, try one new thing. Look for something you wouldn't usually cook, just one, and that week, find out how to cook and eat it.

Always have frozen veg in the freezer. Peas (petit pois are sweeter) and sweetcorn are old freezer staples, but chopped peppers are really convenient for adding to everything from omelettes to pasta sauces. The variety of frozen vegetables available now is amazing, and it means not having to worry about them going off.

Have fresh veg that you know you will always be able to use. I always have carrots (useful for raw snacks, grated on salads or cooked with just about everything) and broccoli (also good raw and cooked in anything from stir fry to steamed on the side) in my fridge. Both keep well and are easy to use.

Find out what you like in a salad. I grew up in a world where salad was a sad slice of iceberg and a wedge of tomato. I like things like rocket and watercress, spiralised veg like beetroot and carrot, edamame beans, grapes, walnuts. People hate salads because some salads are just bad. Try some options.

Veg with breakfast could be: Asparagus to dip in your boiled egg, spinach in your scrambled egg, peppers in your omelette (I like eggs…) Mushrooms on toast (with spinach). Baked beans (they count…) A few tomatoes on the side. A vegetable smoothie.

Veg with lunch could be a side salad, or just a handful of salad in your sandwich or wrap. Raw carrot sticks. A snack pot of edamame beans and other green stuff with dressing. Raw sugar snap peas. Sliced raw pepper.

To increase vegetable intake with dinner, you can think about veg "on the side" like peas, sweetcorn, broccoli, steamed carrot etc, or you can try hidden veg like courgetti (spiralised courgette mixed in with your pasta), grated carrot or diced pepper in stews or pasta sauces. Butternut squash grated goes beautifully into creamy sauces. Frozen spinach is chopped really fine and goes well into pasta sauce or curry, it ends up looking like herbs and you hardly notice it.

If you find it tricky to add a bounteous enough veg portion to a meal, try a veg snack instead.

Some of us feel badly towards vegetables because we are holding onto ideas we have had since childhood - but your tastes change, give it another go. Sometimes it's a struggle because your palate is used to processed foods and sweet things, if that's the case, go in on sugarsnap peas or other sweeter gateway vegetables, you can work towards the other stuff slowly. You don't need to like every vegetable either, just enough to have a nice variety.

You might notice that I haven't mentioned fruit (apart from tomatoes…) here. You are still encouraged to eat fruit as snacks and desserts, but fruit is easy, the goal here is veg. If you have 3 portions of veg and 2 of fruit per day, you are winning your habit and getting your "5 a day".

I often get asked about supplements. There is nothing wrong with taking a multivitamin if you wish to. The current accepted advice is that a good diet should cover all your micronutrient needs, except for Vitamin D in the winter. However, some people do find that a supplement helps them. If you are going to take a supplement a standard multivitamin is fine, don't stack multiple supplements with overlapping ingredients. Omega 3 or fish oil can be helpful, especially if you don't like eating oily fish. Probiotics can be helpful as well. If you suspect you have a deficiency however, you should see a medical professional for diagnosis and treatment.

Eating your vegetables isn't just about micronutrients. While you are eating your meal slowly and mindfully, you will likely notice that vegetables are pretty filling. Between the portion of protein and a fistful of veg, you're going to feel pretty satisfied. This habit is also going to help prevent you from reaching for an extra portion of carbs or an extra snack to fill you up.

Activity

Keep working on your morning flow habit, it's an easy one to slip.

Wellbeing

Finding beauty in new places. We are presented with a very bland and narrow representation of beauty in our culture. Not just in terms of people either. Looking back at fashions in decor, food presentation, even gardening - our cultures constantly shifts the goalposts in terms of what is considered aesthetically desirable. We look back on the hottest trends of years gone by and they have lost their appeal, not because we have learned better, but because our narrow focus has shifted.

The desirable body type is also constantly changing, look at how the women on the catwalk have changed since the days of Cindy Crawford and Naomi Campbell. But not conforming to the current trend doesn't make those women any less beautiful. Current trends don't take away the essence of what caught our eye back then.

The truth is that there is beauty to be found in all kinds of places, not just the places the media directs us. It's there in you, even if you aren't yet prepared to seek or see it.

So your job now is to seek out beauty in quieter places. Take a little time to find some images that you find beautiful. Look at images of

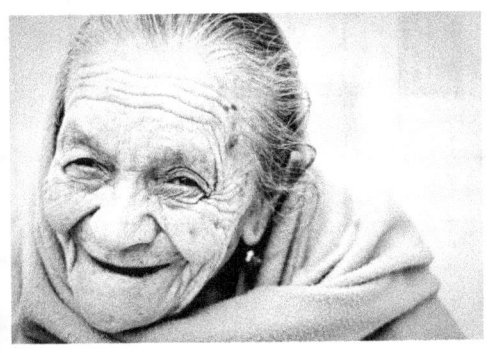

people of a wide variety, and find something beautiful about them, look at images of things that are not people too. You could collect some images on a Pinterest board or similar, so you can add to them and look through them. Look at lots of images of "normal" people. Jade Beall's portraits of mothers are a good example.

Look at images from other cultures. The more we expose ourselves to images of different body types, the more we learn to accept and appreciate those body types, and the yardstick we unconsciously measure ourselves with becomes kinder.

Speaking of kindness, most people with poor self image are able to speak to themselves extremely unkindly, but would never even think such things about the people they care about. So get into the habit of looking at your friends, family - the people you are surrounded by, and find something lovely about them. The habit of looking for beauty, rather than flaws, will gradually creep into how you look at yourself. You might not be ready to look for your own loveliness, but it's not so hard to find it in others.

Your phase 7 checklist

Day	1	2	3	4	5	6	7
Ate a portion of vegetables with each meal							
Started the day with movement							
Appreciated something beautiful							

Phase 8

And we are really storming through it now! Let's keep our focus

You have tried new habits, thought about things that you probably never gave a moment's contemplation to previously. You are managing your life like a boss. You have tried things that made a difference, some that didn't and some that were just plain odd. Check you out, you pioneer of lifestyle science!

Nutrition

This phase we are going to take a look at our calorie dense extras.

Do you find that when you have a really balanced, healthy day of meals, you get to the point where you think "you know what, I could really do with eating a pack of doughnuts, and dammit, I deserve it"? Well, this one's for you.

If you are at all familiar with my work, you will know that I love cake. Cake is my most favourite thing in the whole world. As such, one of the promises I make to anyone I work with is this:

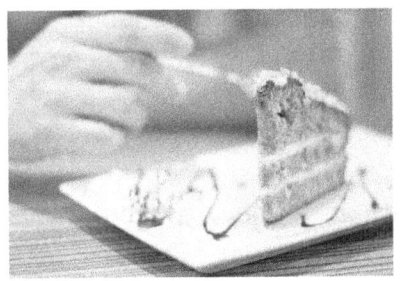

You do not have to give up your favourite "treats".

In fact to do so would be completely in opposition to my ethos of good health, through good living. So how do you have your cake and not sabotage your healthy eating?

Let me share a couple of tricks. Firstly, I work on an 80% rule. For pretty much everything. We hit 80% of our habits on 80% of the days.

We eat until we are 80% full (4 on the hunger scale). Lastly, 80% of our calories come from minimally processed food.

That leaves you 20% for fun.

So on 2000 calories a day, that means I can put aside 400 calories for the sort of stuff that "diets" and "clean eating" tell us we I can't have. Now I don't count calories, so I say it's roughly one treat, or two small treats. It doesn't need to be precise, it just means that while you are prioritising your lean protein, veggies, wholefoods etc, you still have space for a dessert, cake, chocolate bar, whatever tickles your fancy.

Here is my second trick. Be a snob. Go for quality. It's really easy to eat low quality, high calorie foods in large amounts. Good quality treats are much more satisfying. So go for fancy, high cocoa chocolate over the sugar and vegetable oil kind. You'll get the same kick without the compulsion to eat a tonne. Eventually your palate adapts and the cheap stuff isn't so good anymore, but in the meantime, the good stuff is, well, pretty good.

Your habit in this phase is to keep track of your calorie-dense treats, whatever they might be. Desserts, cake, biscuits, savoury snacks. The stuff you might refer to as "junk". It might be a snack, it might be part of a meal. On your checksheet, mark off a tally of how many you are getting in a day.

Your first level here is to just observe. For the first week, don't try to reduce, just see what your intake looks like.

Once you have that down, maybe you've got an average for the week. You might have even noticed a time when you are eating more.

The next level is to try and cut back. Can you do one less a day? Can you do 3 less in the week? If your Friday night is usually binge night, can you just reduce that. Note I say reduce, not eliminate. If your intake is actually quite low already, can you keep it within one per day?

Choose a target which feels attainable to you, based on your current intake.

Activity

This phase, continue to start your day with movement. If you have mastered a morning flow, maybe you can throw in a brisk walk or quick round of tabata before your morning shower?

Wellbeing

You deserve a full life. I'm telling you right now, the pair of jeans you don't fit into is not a reason to stay in and avoid spending time with friends. How you look in a swimming costume should not be stopping you spending time with your kids at the beach. You are allowed to go out for a nice restaurant meal, even if you are overweight. Give yourself permission.

How many things are you putting off "until I lose a bit of weight"? What opportunities are you going to regret missing because you felt your body wasn't "right"? How much fun could you be having at that dance class, if you weren't waiting until you were "fitter"?

We are conditioned to believe that our worth is based on how near or far we are from a given aesthetic. It's lies and it's not going to fly here. You deserve to do fun stuff, wear clothes you feel beautiful in (remember all those kinds of beauty we looked at last phase), and to feel good about yourself.

I'd like you to make a list of things you would like to experience, or do more of, but feel held back because of how you feel about your body.

Take a couple of minutes each day to either add to that list, or to consider how you are going to overcome the barriers. Maybe you'll look for a cute beach outfit for that holiday you've been avoiding. Maybe you'll bite the bullet and just take that dance class, grab a friend for moral support.

Put your list in order, from the easiest to most challenging. Can you do, or arrange one thing a week? Don't wait to start living your awesome future.

Your phase 8 checklist

Day	1	2	3	4	5	6	7
Tally your treats and sweets							
Started the day with movement							
Worked towards your body positive bucket list.							

Phase 9

Welcome to the penultimate stage! Don't slow down though, we are pushing all the way to the finish line!

Nutrition

So how did reducing the calorie dense foods go? OK? Manageable? Getting there?

This week we are going to look at another source of surplus calories that is frankly, easy pickings. Or is it?

High calorie drinks. Some of us drink an awful lot of calories without thinking about it. Some of us simply don't, but it's definitely time to check in on that. So what do I mean by high calorie drinks?

- High sugar carbonated drinks, like cola and lemonade
- Alcoholic drinks
- Fruit juice
- Smoothies
- Milky or sugary coffee

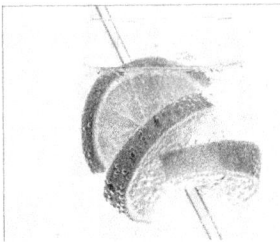

Now I'm not saying all these are bad (no foods are bad) and you should completely avoid them, but if you are struggling to keep your energy intake manageable, it's super easy to gulp down a snack, or even a meal's worth of calories and barely notice it.

Fruit juice or a smoothie can be great as part of a snack, but just for this phase, we are going to experiment with alternatives.

How far you take this might depend, just like the last one, on how much you usually consume. If you are keeping yourself going on a 6 can a day habit of caffeinated high sugar beverage, knocking it off to zero is going to be uncomfortable. But maybe you could try replacing one of those?

So if you are feeling really up for it, sure, make your goal zero high calorie drinks. Knock it on the head and replace them with water, fruit tea, squash, even standard tea or coffee with a splash of milk.
Next level? Try only consuming those drinks as a snack. So have a smoothie and some nuts for your morning snack. Or a latte with a greek yoghurt with some fancy topping. But make it a definite "meal", not simply hydration. Keeping up your glass of water habit should help with this.

If you are a souped up beverage fiend, then start with a tally, just like last week. Work out how much is your "normal" then decide how you could reduce it.

Remember, this is an experiment. See what it feels like to make the change. There's no way I would suggest you should eliminate high calorie drinks forever. This is simply about being aware of how they feature in your day, and making an informed decision about how you would like that to be, going forward.

Activity

Let's check in on moving every hour. How's that going? Can you find new ways to move or new things to do?

Mindset

This phase is about reframing. Reframing is an important mental skill that allows you to be flexible and manage destructive ways of thinking.

When you look at your body, or feel what it is like to inhabit, you will undoubtedly come across things that make you uncomfortable, or that you downright dislike. You might have a habit of standing in front of your mirror and thinking negative things about your body. So far we have looked at refocusing from that - finding a neutral or positive observation to replace it with, but now we are going to start dealing with the trickier stuff.

There's actually 2 stages to this. The first is to be able to sit in discomfort, when we learn that we are able to withstand uncomfortable situations, they become less uncomfortable. We did that when we practiced feeling hungry for a while before eating. Now the uncomfortable feeling is going to be allowing yourself to focus on the things in your body that you perceive as shortcomings. The first stage is to acknowledge it.

Once you have identified the "issue", you get to reframe it. Every "imperfection" on your body is part of your story. Acknowledge it and tell yourself that story in a neutral or positive way. It might be easier to see an example.

I have a large ragged scar from an emergency appendectomy. It tells the story of how I nearly died, but I didn't, and my body was able to rebuild and carry on. It tells of how the surgeon had to carry out an unplanned procedure to treat a condition he didn't believe I had, because I am badass and can function with pain others couldn't bear.

I hate my nose, I always have, but I also know that it's my dad's nose, and even though he has been gone for years, I can just look in the mirror and see part of his face.

Every scar, every stretchmark, every quirk is uniquely a part of you and tells a part of your story. The limitations that you had to find the strength to work around, and those that made you step back and try another path. Every little way you deviate from the ordinary is something you can celebrate as part of what makes you extraordinary.

My body can....

When you are working towards a goal. Even a really healthy one that makes you feel good, sometimes the distance from the goal can highlight things that feel like shortcomings. You end up thinking about what you can't do, and that's not very uplifting.

Striving to reach a goal is great, but let's stop and smell the roses and appreciate how far you have come.

Every day I want you to think of one thing your body can do. It might be something new since starting the programme, it might be something it could already do, or something it accomplished in the past. Write it down and put it somewhere you can see it, on the fridge, on a post it note in your diary, or just make a list under your checklist. Look back at it at the end of a week and see how amazing your body is.

Some ideas:

My body can - walk up the hill to work without stopping to catch my breath.
My body can - lift my children to give them a hug.
My body can - heal when I allow it rest.
My body can - thrive on the good food I've been feeding it.
My body can - keep carrying me, even when it is tired or hurting.
My body can - get stronger when I give it the gift of regular exercise.

Your phase 9 checklist

Day	1	2	3	4	5	6	7
No high calorie drinks							
Moved every hour							
Body positive practice							

Phase 10

Are we nearly there yet?

YES! Yes we are! And also of course, no.

This is a lifelong journey of living well and being the best caretakers for our bodies that we can. With good food, good times and plenty of compassion.

But we are near the end of the programme, for this is the last phase. Well done if you have got this far. By my reckoning it's likely taken you around 5 months, and that's a lot of learning, a lot of practice, and enough time to start to feel, and see, some real changes.

Nutrition

It makes sense that our last habit is going to be one that we will be working on in the long term. It's this :

Eat as much as you can in its minimally processed form.

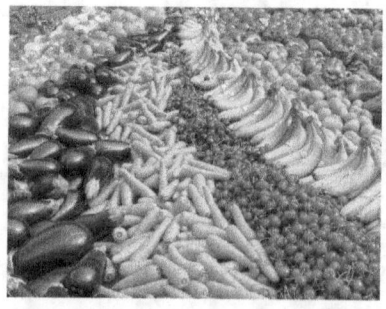

Back in Phase 7, we did vegetable eating, where we started to incorporate more colourful veggies. Prepared in a variety of ways.

We've also done lean proteins, which tend to be fairly unprocessed because, well, that's how they come.

We've downsized our calorically dense treat foods and drinks, which by their nature tend to be highly processed.

In reality, you are well on the way.

This is going to be an ongoing theme, because this, even as the last habit is one of the real cornerstones of a healthy diet. You don't have to forgo all processed foods, remember the 80% rule? That's a good start. We also don't need to quibble about what "processed" means.

Just aim to make a choice for the option that looks like, well, what it is. How you play this out is up to you, and remember, we aren't going for perfect, just a little bit better, every day.

I think now is a good time to remind ourselves of the foundation of healthy, intuitive, habit based eating, let's go for it....

- Eat when you are hungry, in the belly
- Eat slowly and with awareness.
- Stop eating when you are satisfied, not stuffed.
- Eat a portion of lean protein with every meal.
- Eat a portion of colourful vegetables with every meal.
- Drink water, regularly.
- Make the majority of your diet minimally processed.

And that is all there is. Stick to those rules and your body will regulate your eating and manage your weight. Easy right? Well I hope it seems easier now. It might not have been in the beginning, but we've come a long way, building the skills to do this, you are ready now.

Activity

We are going to leave off by going back to basics. We've worked on a lot of different elements to do with this movement business, but what it still boils down to is move, be active. So take whatever parts of the practice you have enjoyed and keep doing them. Maybe find new things to try and play with. Keep moving for 30 minutes a day.

Wellbeing

Sleep

Just like the other habits, our journey with sleep has been about trying out things that might work for you. Whether it's working out your best bedtime (and perhaps waking time), finding your best wind-down routine or pacing yourself through the day. Keep practicing the routine that works for you, and continue to aim for 7-9 hours of sleep for adequate rest and recovery.

Stress

This is your life now. Hopefully introducing a stress management practice has helped you to integrate stress management, rest and recovery into your life. Keep going, it will add productivity to your day, clarity to your thoughts and years to your life.

Mindset

Now we are heading towards the end, I'm hoping you are finding it easier to think in more positive terms about your body and capabilities.

You've taken time to accept your body as it is. You have considered what your body can do and the stories it holds. Take time to notice changes that came from caring for your body through healthy eating, mindful rest and movement.

This phase I would like you to come up with a daily statement about your body or health, that is positive in nature.

What can you find to like or enjoy about being you, in the body you have today? Anything you like. Take a deep breath and think about what feels good. Think about the things you did today that your body carried you through. Think about the parts of your body that you like, or are learning to like.

I want you to work on your body positive mindset, with daily mindfulness of the awesomeness that you are piloting around your life. Be aware of all the great stuff your body can do, even right this second as your ridiculously complex network of cells and chemical soup detect these words and figure out their meanings.

You've come a long way from stage one. I'm proud of you.

Keep learning to love yourself, and when you are ready, let that shine, show those around you how love themselves and treat themselves (and others) with compassion.

Your Free Living checklist

Day	1	2	3	4	5	6	7
Ate roughly 80% minimally processed							

foods.							
30 minutes of activity a day							
7-9 hours of restful sleep							
5 minutes stress management							
Body positive practice							

So this is goodbye

Thank you for choosing to come along on this journey with me. I hope it has been enjoyable, or at least (in the tougher parts) interesting. I hope you have learned a little bit more about what you are capable of, in mind and body. I hope you have found new things you enjoy, and maybe some things you know not to try again!

For some people, the journey to good health and habits can be rougher. If you feel you need more guidance, a hand to hold, or extra help overcoming obstacles that are specific to you, then please don't hesitate to get in touch.

You'll find all my contact details, up to date social media etc at www.firelotusfitness.com. I am always happy to have a chat, and I also offer personalised, one to one coaching for nutrition and habit change.

I wish you a bright and healthy future.

Appendices

Your Food and Mood diary

	6-9am	9-12	12-3pm	3-6pm	6-9pm	9-12
Day 1 Food						
Hunger before/ after						
Mood						
Day 2 Food						
Hunger before/ after						
Mood						
Day 3 Food						
Hunger before/						

	6-9am	9-12	12-3pm	3-6pm	6-9pm	9-12
after						
Mood						

	6-9am	9-12	12-3pm	3-6pm	6-9pm	9-12
Day 4 Food						
Hunger before/ after						
Mood						
Day 5 Food						
Hunger before/ after						
Mood						
Day 6 Food						

Hunger before/ after						
Mood						
Day 7 Food						
Hunger before/ after						
Mood						

Your Phase 1 checklist

Day	1	2	3	4	5	6	7
Updated my food and mood diary							

Completed 30 minutes of activity today							
5 minutes stress management							

Your Phase 2 checklist

Day	1	2	3	4	5	6	7
Ate 3-4 times in the day							
30 minutes walking or light activity							
Neutral self talk							

Your Phase 3 checklist

Day	1	2	3	4	5	6	7
Waited 30 minutes hungry before eating							

Moved around for 5 minutes 6 times during the day						
Went to bed on time						

Your Phase 4 checklist

Day	1	2	3	4	5	6	7
Ate 3 portions of protein							
Moved around for 5 minutes 6 times during the day							
Practiced bedtime routine							

Your phase 5 checklist

Day	1	2	3	4	5	6	7
Ate one meal slowly, and stopped when satisfied							
Started the day with movement							
Got up on the first alarm							

Your phase 6 checklist

Day	1	2	3	4	5	6	7
Drank a glass of water with each meal and workout							
Started the day with movement							
Daily act of self care							

Your phase 7 checklist

Day	1	2	3	4	5	6	7
Ate a portion of vegetables with each meal							
Started the day with movement							
Appreciated something beautiful							

Your phase 8 checklist

Day	1	2	3	4	5	6	7
Tally your treats and sweets							
Started the day with movement							
Worked towards your body positive bucket list.							

Your phase 9 checklist

Day	1	2	3	4	5	6	7
No high calorie drinks							
Moved every hour							
Body positive practice							

Your Free Living checklist

Day	1	2	3	4	5	6	7
Ate roughly 80% minimally processed foods.							
30 minutes of activity a day							
7-9 hours of restful sleep							
5 minutes stress management							
Body positive practice							

A sample from the Free Living Fitness Daily Planner

WEDNESDAY

DATE: ....

IMPORTANT TASKS

EXERCISE AND ACTIVITY

HABIT PRACTICES

TODAY'S BIG WIN

FOOD DIARY

MORNING

Hunger before   1 2 3 4 5

Hunger after   1 2 3 4 5

AFTERNOON

Hunger before   1 2 3 4 5

Hunger after   1 2 3 4 5

EVENING

Hunger before   1 2 3 4 5

Hunger after   1 2 3 4 5

SNACKS

Hunger before   1 2 3 4 5

Hunger after   1 2 3 4 5

READY FOR TOMORROW

About the author

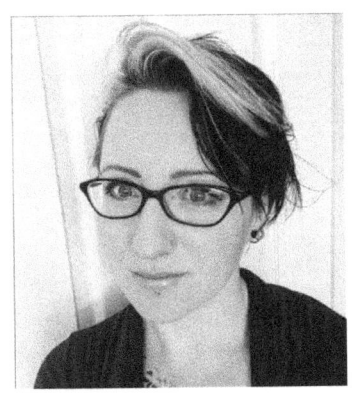

Claire Hunter is a Personal Trainer, Precision Nutrition Certified Coach, Bellydancer, Yogi, Doula, Powerlifter and defender of all that is awesome and has yet to realise it.

Claire is spreading the message the health and fitness should be fun, accessible and empowering for everyone.

Claire is based in Glastonbury, Somerset, surrounded by small boys and chickens. She provides online coaching and programming to people all over the world.

Find her at www.firelotusfitness.com